INTERMITTENT FASTING FOR WOMEN OVER 50.

A Comprehensive Guide To Discovering The Power Of Intermittent Fasting As A Means To Revitalising Aging.

Larisa Charlie

Table of Contents.

INTRODUCTION

As we journey through life, our bodies undergo profound changes, especially during the second half of our lives. Women over 50 often experience shifts in metabolism, hormonal balance, and overall body composition, which can sometimes feel like an uphill battle against time. However, within these pages, we will explore a revolutionary approach to wellness that holds the power to rewrite the rules of aging.

Intermittent fasting has gained a lot of attention in recent years as a popular weight-loss and health-promoting strategy. It involves alternating periods of fasting and non-fasting, which can lead to numerous benefits for the body and mind. While the concept of intermittent fasting may seem intimidating at first, it is becoming increasingly popular among women over 50 who are looking for a sustainable and effective way to maintain their health and well-being. This book is designed specifically for women over 50 who are interested in intermittent fasting and want to learn more about how it can help them achieve their health goals. It also addresses FAQs about intermittent fasting.

By embracing the power of intermittent fasting, you have the opportunity to redefine your relationship with food, nurture self-care practices, and cultivate a newfound sense of empowerment that permeates every aspect of your life.

Whether you are new to fasting or have been practicing it for some time, this book will provide you with valuable insights, tips, and strategies to help you make the most of intermittent fasting and live your best life.

UNDERSTANDING INTERMITTENT FASTING

I. Definition Of Intermittent Fasting.

Intermittent fasting is a dietary practice that involves alternating between fasting and eating windows of time. It places more emphasis on when to eat than what to eat. Depending on the fasting strategy that is adopted, the periods of fasting might last anywhere from a few hours to a whole day or longer. No calories or very few calories are taken during the fasting periods, allowing the body to enter a state of metabolic rest and cellular repair.

Instead of focusing on altering the timing of meals, intermittent fasting is not a diet that restricts dietary choices. It is a flexible approach to healthy eating because it can be modified to suit individual preferences and time constraints. The 16/8 technique, which involves fasting for 16 hours and eating every meal within an 8-hour window, and the 5:2 approach, which involves five days of regular eating followed by two days where calorie intake is limited to a certain number, are examples of popular fasting strategies.

The main objective of intermittent fasting is to enhance metabolic functions and advance a number of health advantages. It is possible to lose weight and improve body composition by lengthening the fasting period because the body uses energy that is stored, largely in fat cells. Furthermore, intermittent fasting has been linked to a number of positive health effects, such as increased insulin sensitivity, decreased inflammation, greater cellular repair, and possible advantages for longevity and brain function.

It is important to remember that not everyone should practice intermittent fasting, particularly those with certain medical conditions, women who are pregnant, nursing, or underweight.

Before beginning any fasting regimen, it is advised to speak with a healthcare practitioner to make sure it is in line with the needs and goals of the individual.

II. How Does Intermittent Fasting work.

When you fast, your body starts using fat and glucose that have been stored as energy. A fast can help your body burn fat for energy because it lowers insulin levels. Furthermore, fasting may increase the flow of human growth hormone (HGH), which can support muscular growth and fat metabolism in your body.

Numerous health advantages of intermittent fasting have been demonstrated, including lower inflammation, increased insulin sensitivity, weight loss, and enhanced cognitive performance. Additionally, it might offer some degree of defense against certain chronic conditions like cancer, heart disease, and type 2 diabetes.

Intermittent fasting is not a miracle cure for weight loss or good health, it is important to remember this. It's just one of the tools that can be utilized in conjunction with a healthy diet and way of living to improve your overall well-being.

III. Benefits Of Intermittent Fasting For Women Over 50.

While intermittent fasting has gained popularity due to its possible health benefits, it is vital to evaluate how it may affect specific groups, such as women over the age of 50. Intermittent fasting can assist women of this age maintain their general well-being while also improving certain parts of their health. Let us look at some of these advantages:

Weight management: Because of hormonal changes and a slower metabolism, women's weight management might become more difficult as they age. Intermittent fasting can be an effective weight-management method for women over 50. Intermittent fasting, by limiting the eating window, can help reduce calorie intake and enhance fat loss, resulting in better weight control.

Insulin sensitivity and blood sugar regulation: Intermittent fasting has been proven to improve insulin sensitivity, which is vital for maintaining stable blood sugar levels. Intermittent fasting can lessen the risk of getting type 2 diabetes and help manage existing blood sugar abnormalities by boosting insulin sensitivity. This benefit is especially important for women over 50, who may be predisposed to insulin resistance and other health difficulties.

Hormonal balance: Hormonal changes during menopause can cause a variety of symptoms such as hot flashes, mood swings, and sleep difficulties. Intermittent fasting has been shown to improve hormonal balance.Some studies have found that intermittent fasting can help with hormone balance, perhaps relieving menopausal symptoms and enhancing overall well-being in women over 50.

Cardiovascular health: Because the risk of heart disease grows with age, women over 50 ought to pay close attention to their cardiovascular health. Intermittent fasting has been shown to improve a variety of cardiovascular health indices, including blood pressure reduction, improved cholesterol profiles, and decreased triglyceride levels. These advantages can help women over 50 have a healthier heart and lower their risk of cardiovascular disease.

Cognitive Functioning: Aging is frequently related with cognitive impairment and an increased risk of neurological disorders like Alzheimer's. According to new research, intermittent fasting may have neuroprotective effects and benefit brain health. Intermittent fasting may improve cognitive performance and protect against age-related cognitive decline in women over 50 by lowering oxidative stress and inflammation.

Longevity and cellular health: Intermittent fasting has been related to improved longevity and cell wellness. Animal studies have indicated that intermittent fasting can boost cellular repair mechanisms, reduce oxidative damage, and increase overall longevity. While additional research is needed to properly understand the effects of intermittent fasting on human lifespan, these findings suggest that it may promote healthy aging in women older than 50.

It is important to note that intermittent fasting may not be appropriate for everyone, and particular concerns, such as pre-existing medical conditions or medications, should be considered. Before making any significant dietary changes, women over the age of 50 should consult with a healthcare expert.

Nonetheless, when done correctly and under professional supervision, intermittent fasting has the potential to provide significant health benefits for women in this age group, boosting their general health and well-being.

IV. Common Misconceptions About Intermittent Fasting.

Intermittent fasting has received a lot of attention in recent years, but with it has come a lot of misconceptions and misunderstandings. Let's clarify some prevalent myths about intermittent fasting:

Intermittent fasting means starving yourself: It is a prevalent misperception that intermittent fasting equates to starving. However, intermittent fasting does not imply deprivation of food. It is a methodical practice that alternates between eating and fasting periods. During the eating window, you consume the calories and nutrients your body needs to function efficiently.

Intermittent fasting causes muscle loss: One common concern is that intermittent fasting could cause muscle loss. Intermittent fasting, if done properly, should not result in considerable muscle loss. In fact, research has shown that combining intermittent fasting with resistance training can help to preserve muscle mass and even increase muscular growth. To support muscle health, it's important to eat a well-balanced diet and exercise regularly, as well as practice intermittent fasting.

Intermittent fasting is only about weight loss: Weight loss is one of the potential benefits of intermittent fasting, but it is not the only one. Other benefits of intermittent fasting include increased insulin sensitivity, greater cellular repair mechanisms, improved cardiovascular health, and cognitive benefits. Weight loss is only one part of the full range of potential benefits of intermittent fasting.

Intermittent fasting means skipping breakfast: Skipping breakfast is a common method in various intermittent fasting protocols; however, skipping breakfast is not the only way to practise intermittent fasting. There are other approaches, such as the 16/8 strategy, which involves fasting for 16 hours and having an 8-hour eating window that may be altered to suit individual preferences. Intermittent fasting can be tailored to fit various schedules and lifestyles.

Intermittent fasting is suitable for everyone: While intermittent fasting can benefit many people, it may not be appropriate for everyone. Before beginning an intermittent fasting routine, any individual with certain medical issues, such as diabetes, eating disorders, or hormonal imbalances, ought to apply caution or speak with a healthcare expert. Women who are pregnant or breastfeeding may need to take precaution whilst fasting since their nutritional demands vary.

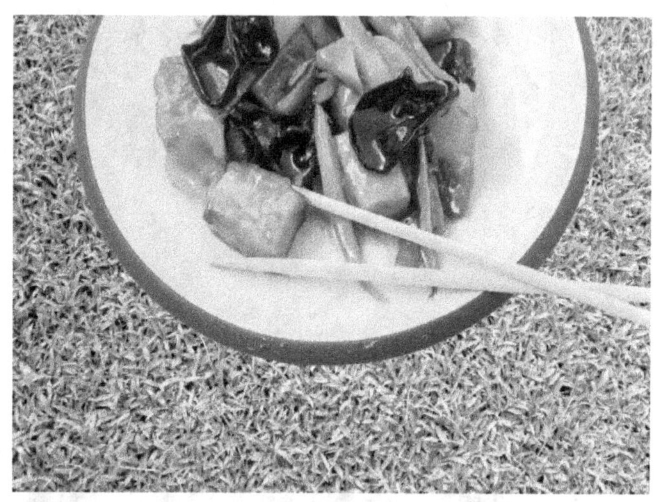

Intermittent fasting means unrestricted eating during the eating window: It is important to understand that intermittent fasting is not an authorization to eat unhealthy foods during the eating window.For the sake of your overall wellness, the focus should remain on eating a well-balanced, nutrient-dense diet. To maximize the benefits of intermittent fasting, choose nutritious foods, lean meats, fruits and vegetables, and healthy fats.

As with any nutritional strategy, it's important to approach intermittent fasting with understanding, listen to your body, and make adjustments based on individual needs and preferences.

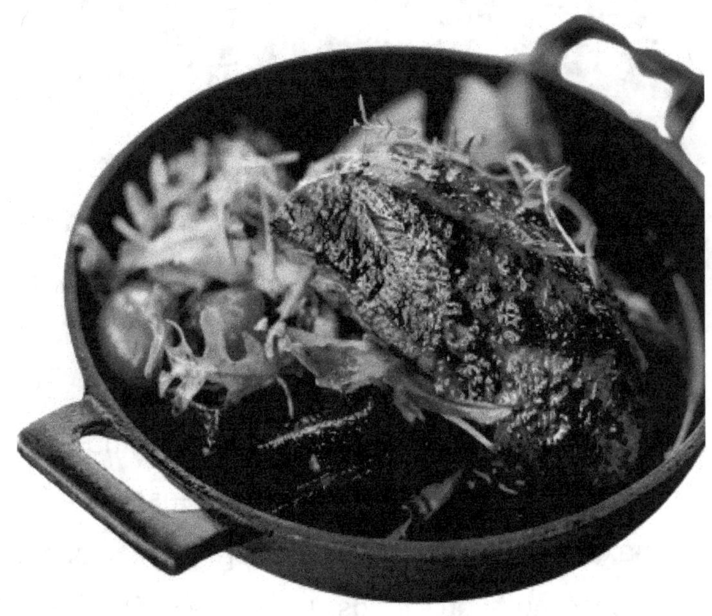

18

THE AGING PROCESS AND NUTRITION CHANGES

I. Changes In The Body With Age.

Our bodies experience lots of changes as we age . While these changes can differ from person to person, there are some common changes that take place as we age. Here are some noticeable transformations that the body undergoes as it ages:

Skin: The skin changes are among the most noticeable. Age spots, fine lines, and wrinkles develop as a result of the gradual loss of suppleness and thinning of our skin as we get older. Over time, the amount of collagen and elastin produced, which keep the skin elastic and tight, diminishes. These changes can happen more quickly if you engage in certain lifestyle choices, like smoking, or are exposed to environmental causes, like sun damage.

Muscle and bones: Muscle mass and strength naturally drop as we age, a condition known as sarcopenia. Mobility, balance, and general physical performance could all be affected as a result of this muscle loss. In addition, bone density declines, increasing the risk of fractures and osteoporosis, especially in postmenopausal women.

Joints: Over time, the joints in our body, such as the knees, hips, and shoulders, start showing signs of wear and strain. As a result, disorders like osteoarthritis may develop and cause stiffness and a reduction in range of motion. As we age, we may experience increasing joint pain and stiffness.

Cardiovascular system: Changes are also experienced by the cardiovascular system. Blood arteries may stiffen and lose some of their flexibility, which can raise blood pressure and increase the risk of heart disease. The cardiac muscle may become slightly thicker and less effective at pumping. Reduced overall cardiovascular function could potentially be the result of these changes.

Metabolism: Aging generally causes a slowdown in metabolism. Thus, the body expends fewer calories while at rest, making weight management more difficult. Losing muscle mass and a slowing metabolism can both lead to weight gain and a higher chance of developing diseases like diabetes.

Hormonal changes: In women especially, hormonal changes are a normal aspect of aging. Menopause signals the end of the reproductive years and results in a drop in estrogen and progesterone levels. It commonly happens in women in their late 40s to early 50s. Hot flashes, mood swings, and changes in bone density are just a few of the symptoms that can result from this hormonal imbalance.

Sensory changes: As we age, our senses also change. The chance of developing illnesses like cataracts and glaucoma rises, and vision may become less precise. Another typical age-related change is hearing loss, especially in higher frequencies. Sensitivity to smell and taste may also deteriorate.

While these changes are a natural part of aging, maintaining a healthy lifestyle can help lessen their impact. Regular exercise, a healthy diet, adequate hydration, and skincare routines can all help improve your overall well-being and reduce the progression of certain age-related changes. Regular check-ups with healthcare specialists can also help in the early detection and management of age-related conditions.

II. Nutritional Needs For Women Over 50; Foods To Include and Avoid.

Women's dietary demands change as they age, so it's vital to focus on overall health while also addressing specific concerns that may occur with age. Some major nutritional factors for women over 50 include:

Calories: Because women's metabolic rates tend to slow as they age, they may require fewer calories. Individual calorie needs, on the other hand, are determined by characteristics such as activity level, body composition, and overall health.

Protein is essential for muscle mass maintenance, bone health, and general vitality. Protein foods that are low in fat and calories include poultry, fish, beans, lentils, tofu, and Greek yogurt.

Calcium and Vitamin D: As women age, bone health becomes a major concern, making adequate calcium and vitamin D intake critical. Dairy products, fortified plant-based milks, leafy greens, and fortified cereals are all calcium-rich foods. Vitamin D can be gained through sunlight or dietary sources such as fatty fish, fortified dairy products, and supplements if needed.

Fiber: Adequate fiber intake is necessary for digestive health, bowel regularity, and weight management. To meet your fiber needs, include low-glycemic fruits like berries, apples, pears, and citrus fruits. They are lower in sugar and high in fiber, providing essential nutrients and antioxidants. Colorful vegetables such as broccoli, spinach, kale, bell peppers, carrots, and Brussels sprouts. They are packed with vitamins, minerals, and antioxidants. Whole grain options like quinoa, brown rice, oats, and whole wheat bread instead of refined grains. They provide more fiber and nutrients.

Omega-3 Fatty Acids: Omega-3 fatty acids have been linked to improved cardiovascular health and cognitive function. To gain these benefits, include healthy fats like avocados, fatty fish (such as salmon and mackerel), nuts, seeds like flax seeds, Chia seeds and olive oil in your diet.

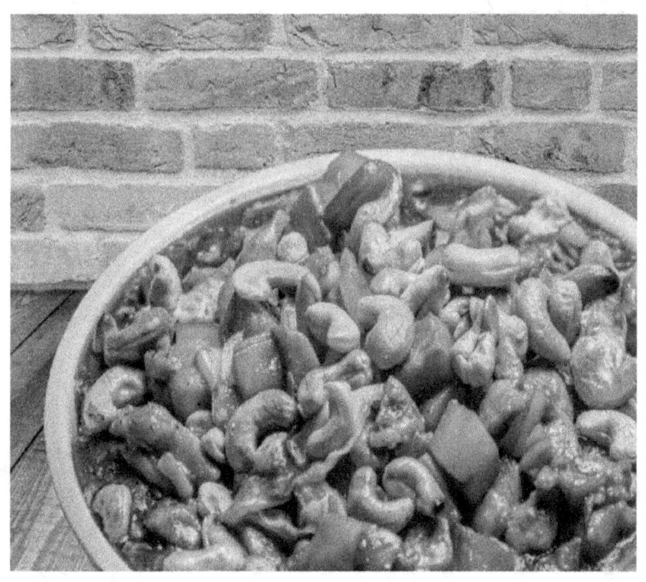

Iron: Although iron requirements may decrease after menopause, it is still important to check iron levels because deficiencies could arise. Lean meats, poultry, fish, fortified cereals, legumes, and leafy green vegetables are all high in iron.

Fluid intake: Everyone, regardless of age, needs to stay hydrated. Drink plenty of water and eat hydrating meals like fruits, vegetables, and soups. You can include herbal teas and infused water for variety.

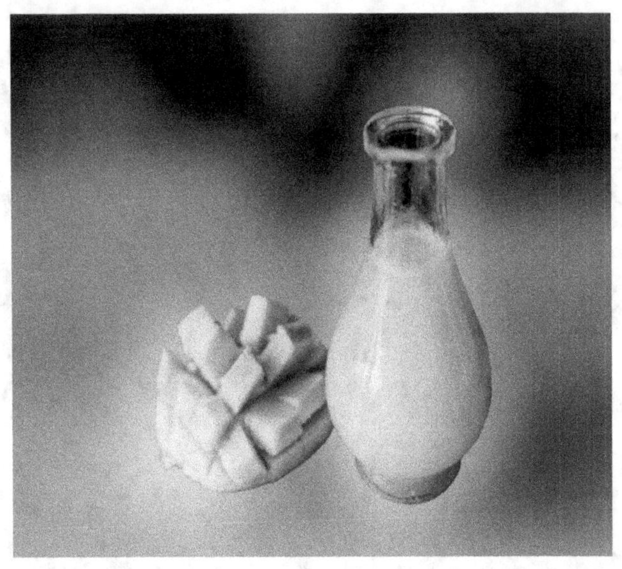

While there is no precise list of items that women over 50 should avoid when fasting, there are some basic rules to follow. Here are a few things to consider :

- Regardless of age or gender, it's typically a good idea to avoid or restrict overly processed foods. Fast food, sugary snacks, packaged snacks, and refined grains are examples of these. When possible, choose whole, unprocessed meals.

- Reduce your intake of sugary foods and beverages, such as soda, sweets, pastries, and sweetened drinks. These can cause weight gain and have an impact on blood sugar levels.

- While healthy fats are a vital component of a balanced diet, it's also important to keep your overall calorie consumption in mind, especially if weight loss is a goal. High-fat foods should be consumed in moderation, such as fried dishes, fatty meats, full-fat dairy products, and butter.

- During your fasting periods, limit your alcohol consumption or avoid it entirely. Alcoholic beverages are high in calories and may interfere with intermittent fasting goals.

- Pay attention to portion sizes, especially if you're trying to lose weight.

III. Choosing The Right Intermittent Fasting Plan.

A few popular intermittent fasting methods to consider are:

Eating on a Time Limit: Time-restricted eating, like the **16/8 technique** or the **14/10 method.** The 16/8 technique entails fasting for 16 hours and limiting your eating window to 8 hours each day. For example, you may skip breakfast and begin eating at noon, then finish by 8 p.m. This method is simple to implement and can fit into the everyday lives of the majority. The duration can be changed to suit your needs as with the 14/10 method which is setting it to a 14-hour fast and a 10-hour eating window.

5:2 Fasting: On the 5:2 diet, you eat normally five days a week and limit your calorie intake to 500-600 calories on the other two days. These two days should not be on the same day. This strategy may suit those who prefer occasional fasting over daily fasting.

Eat-Stop-Eat: This strategy requires a 24-hour fast once or twice a week. For example, you might have dinner on Monday and then not on Tuesday. This strategy may require more discipline and preparation, but it can be efficient for some people.

Alternate-Day Fasting: As the name implies, alternate-day fasting requires you to fast every other day. On fasting days, you may consume extremely few calories (about 500-600) or go completely without food. You eat regularly on non-fasting days. Because of the many fasting days, this strategy may be difficult for certain people.

When selecting an intermittent fasting plan,

- Choose a strategy that works with your daily schedule, work schedule, and social obligations. confirm that it is sustainable over time.

- Contact your healthcare provider if you have any underlying health disorders or concerns. Certain situations may necessitate adjustments or modifications to the fasting strategy.

- Choose an approach that is suitable for your food preferences and eating habits. If you have difficulty fasting for long periods of time, shorter fasting windows or modified approaches may be more suitable.

- Consider your specific goals, such as weight loss, metabolic health, or overall well-being. Some intermittent fasting approaches may be more appropriate for specific aims.

Experiment with different fasting methods to find what works best for you. Bear in mind that intermittent fasting is not suitable for everyone, including pregnant or breastfeeding women, people with a history of eating problems, and people with certain medical conditions.

IV. Incorporating Other Diets Into Intermittent Fasting.

-Low-carb/Ketogenic Diets

A ketogenic diet is a very low-carb, high-fat (healthy fat) diet that tries to release a metabolic condition known as ketosis. In this state, the body's primary source of fuel is ketones, which is produced through fat breakdown. To achieve ketosis, carbohydrate intake is severely limited (typically less than 50 grams per day), while fat intake is increased. This diet typically has considerable protein consumption.

Combining intermittent fasting with a low-carb or ketogenic diet may have a number of benefits:

- Increased Fat burning: By limiting carbohydrate consumption and extending the fasting period, the body is encouraged to use stored fat for fuel, resulting in greater fat burning and probable weight loss.

- Improved Blood Sugar Control: Both low-carb and ketogenic diets have been found to enhance insulin sensitivity and blood sugar level stability, which can be good for people with diabetes or insulin resistance.

- Enhanced Satiety: Consuming the right amount of protein and healthy fats during the eating window can boost satiety and help regulate hunger, making fasting easier to adhere to.

- Mental Clarity and Energy: Many people experience greater mental clarity and sustained energy levels during fasting, which can boost attention and productivity.

-Vegan/Vegetarian Diets

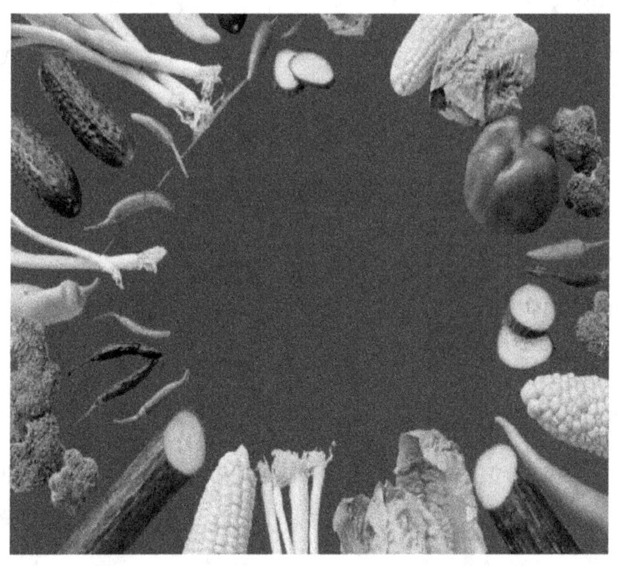

To reach your health and dietary goals, vegan and vegetarian diets can be basically integrated with intermittent fasting. Intermittent fasting is a type of eating habit that alternates between periods of fasting and eating. It does not stipulate what foods you should eat, therefore you can easily practise intermittent fasting while being vegan or vegetarian. Here are some suggestions for combining these two dietary approaches:

Nutrient Balance: It's important to receive all of the nutrients you need when eating a vegan or vegetarian diet. Consume a wide range of plant-based foods, such as fruits, vegetables, legumes, whole grains, nuts, and seeds. This will assist you in meeting your macronutrient (carbohydrates, protein, and fat) as well as micronutrient (vitamins and minerals) requirements.

Protein sources: As a vegan or vegetarian, it's important to monitor your protein consumption during intermittent fasting. Legumes (e.g., lentils, chickpeas, beans), tofu, tempeh, seitan, edamame, quinoa, and certain whole grains are high in protein. These protein sources will help you retain muscle mass while also increasing satiety.

Nutrient-dense meals: To maximise your nutritional intake, focus on eating whole, nutrient-dense foods within your eating window. Include a variety of fresh fruits and vegetables, whole grains, and healthy fats in your diet. This will give you important vitamins, minerals, and fibre while also keeping you full during fasting periods.

Hydration: Drink plenty of water throughout the day, even when fasting. Water, herbal teas, and calorie-free beverages can help reduce appetite and improve overall health.

Remember to listen to your body and make necessary changes to your dietary habits. Pay attention to how you feel and perform during fasting periods, and make any necessary changes to your vegan or vegetarian diet.

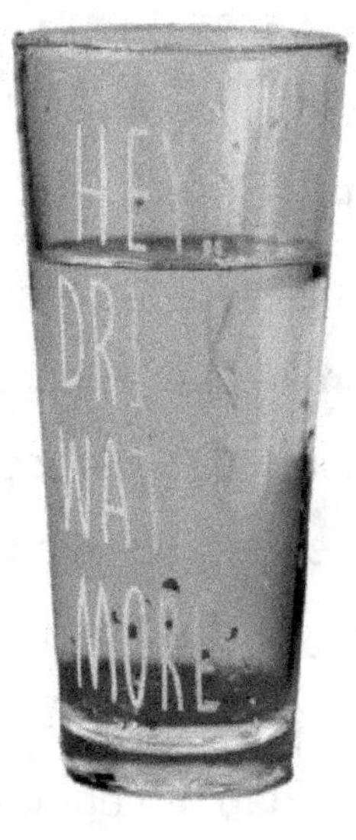

HEY
DRI
WAT
MORE

INTERMITTENT FASTING AND HEALTH CONDITIONS

I. How Intermittent Fasting May Affect Menopause symptoms.

Menopause is a natural biological process that occurs between the ages of 45 and 55 and signals the end of a woman's reproductive years. Hot flashes, mood swings, sleep difficulties, weight gain, and metabolic changes are all signs of menopause. While hormonal changes are the main trigger of menopause symptoms, lifestyle variables such as nutrition can have an impact on symptom intensity.
Some of the potential effects of intermittent fasting on menopause symptoms include:

Weight control: In certain studies, intermittent fasting has been proven to promote weight loss and improve body composition. Because weight gain is typical during menopause, keeping a healthy weight may help relieve symptoms like joint discomfort, hot flashes, and sleep difficulties.

Inflammation: According to some research, intermittent fasting may have anti-inflammatory properties. Inflammation has been linked to a number of menopausal symptoms, including joint discomfort, mood swings, and cognitive loss. Intermittent fasting may help reduce these symptoms by lowering inflammation.

Intermittent fasting has been researched for its influence on insulin and other metabolic markers, but its direct effect on sex hormone levels during menopause is unknown. Menopause is marked by a decrease in oestrogen and progesterone levels, and it is unknown if intermittent fasting impacts these hormone levels or the severity of associated symptoms.

Before beginning any new diet or fasting regimen, it is best to contact your healthcare provider, especially if you have any underlying health disorders or menopausal concerns. Furthermore, a well-balanced diet with adequate nutrients is essential during menopause to maintain general health and well-being.

II. Diabetes And Insulin Resistance.

When you fast, especially for an extended period of time, your insulin levels drop. This insulin decrease promotes the breakdown of stored fatty acids and carbohydrates for energy. This can lead to greater insulin sensitivity over time, which means your body becomes more responsive to insulin, allowing it to properly regulate blood sugar levels and minimize your chance of developing diabetes. Intermittent fasting can reduce the amount of hours your body is exposed to high glucose levels by limiting the duration of eating windows, preventing excessive insulin spikes. This is especially helpful for people who have prediabetes or type 2 diabetes since it helps to stabilize blood sugar levels and improve overall glycemic control. Intermittent fasting can help with weight loss and management, which is important for people. Intermittent fasting can help with weight loss and control, which is especially important for people who have diabetes or insulin resistance. Intermittent fasting can create an energy deficit and promote fat loss by reducing meal frequency and calorie intake during fasting periods. This can result in weight loss, a lower risk of obesity-related insulin resistance, and better metabolic health.

The development and progression of diabetes and insulin resistance are linked to chronic inflammation and oxidative damage. Intermittent fasting has anti-inflammatory and antioxidant benefits, which may contribute to its beneficial effect on these disorders. Fasting increases autophagy, a system that clears away damaged cells and promotes overall cellular health.

III. Heart Disease And High Blood Pressure.

It is important to highlight that research in this field is still evolving, and individual outcomes may vary. However, some research suggests that intermittent fasting may be beneficial for heart disease and high blood pressure. Obesity raises the risk of heart disease and hypertension. Intermittent fasting may help lessen the strain on the heart and lower blood pressure by enhancing weight loss. Chronic inflammation contributes to the development of cardiovascular disease and hypertension. According to certain research, intermittent fasting may help reduce inflammation indicators in the body, which may benefit cardiovascular health.

Also, intermittent fasting has also been shown to improve lipid profiles by lowering LDL cholesterol (commonly referred to as "bad" cholesterol) and triglycerides while boosting HDL cholesterol (typically referred to as "good" cholesterol). A good lipid profile is essential for heart health and blood pressure regulation.

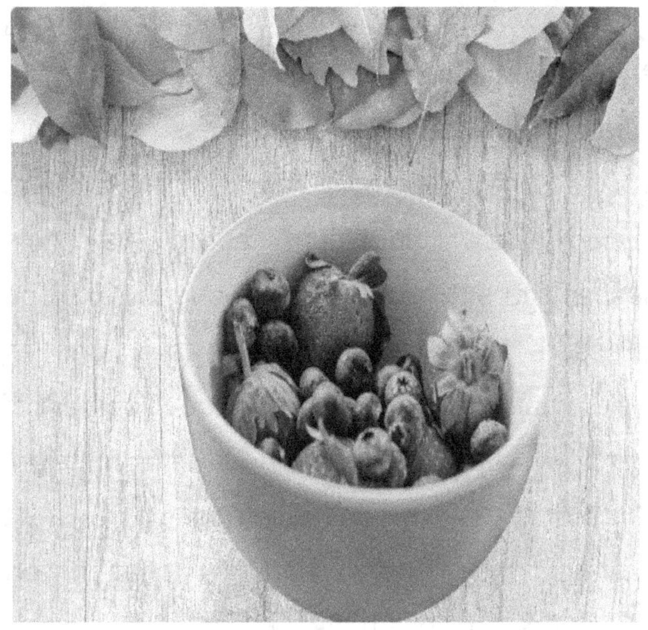

EXERCISE AND INTERMITTENT FASTING

I. Benefits Of Exercising For Aging Women.

Regular exercise has various advantages for elderly ladies. Here are some significant benefits:

Maintains a healthy weight: Physical activity on a regular basis helps to prevent weight gain and promotes weight management. This is especially important for older women since maintaining a healthy weight helps lower the risk of chronic diseases such as heart disease, diabetes, and some cancers.

Enhances cardiovascular health: Aerobic exercise, such as brisk walking, swimming, or cycling, improves heart and lung function, lowers the risk of cardiovascular disease, lowers blood pressure, and improves overall cardiovascular health.

Strengthens bones and muscles: Aging is associated with a decrease in bone density, which contributes to the risk of osteoporosis and fractures. Weight-bearing exercises, resistance training, and activities such as yoga can help improve bone density, muscle mass, and strength, lowering the risk of falls and fractures.

Promotes joint flexibility and mobility: Regular exercise helps preserve joint flexibility and mobility by reducing stiffness. It can help to relieve arthritis symptoms and improve everyday activities, boosting independence and quality of life.

Enhances mental health: Exercise has been shown to improve mental health by releasing endorphins, which are natural mood boosters. Physical activity on a regular basis lowers the chances of depression, anxiety, and stress. It can also boost cognitive function and memory, lowering the chances of age-related cognitive decline.

Improves sleep quality: Sleep problems are common as people age. Regular exercise has been shown to improve sleep quality, allowing older women to get more rest, boost energy levels, and promote general well-being.

Reduces the risk of chronic diseases: Exercise is essential in the prevention of chronic diseases such as heart disease, type 2 diabetes, certain cancers, and stroke. Regular physical activity can considerably reduce the risk of many diseases by boosting general health and well-being.

Improves balance and lowers the risk of falling: Balance activities, such as tai chi, can enhance balance and stability, lowering the risk of falls and associated injuries. This is especially significant for aged women who may be more prone to falling due to muscle weakness or balance concerns.

Boosts social interaction: Participating in group exercise courses or activities increases opportunities for social interaction and promotes a sense of community. This can help older persons overcome feelings of isolation and loneliness.

Increases overall longevity: Exercise has been linked to a longer lifespan in studies. Exercise can help elderly women live longer, healthier lives by increasing general health and lowering the risk of chronic diseases.

II. Best Exercises To Combine With Intermittent Fasting.

Resistance Training: Including strength training exercises, such as weightlifting or bodyweight exercises, in your workout routine helps you grow and retain muscle mass while shedding fat.

HIIT (High-Intensity Interval Training): HIIT workouts consist of short bursts of intensive activity followed by rest intervals. They are both time-efficient and effective at burning calories and improving cardiovascular fitness.

Cardiovascular exercise, such as brisk walking, jogging, cycling, or swimming, can increase calorie expenditure while also supporting general health and weight management.

Yoga or Pilates: These activities improve flexibility, balance, and core strength while also improving your general health and well-being.

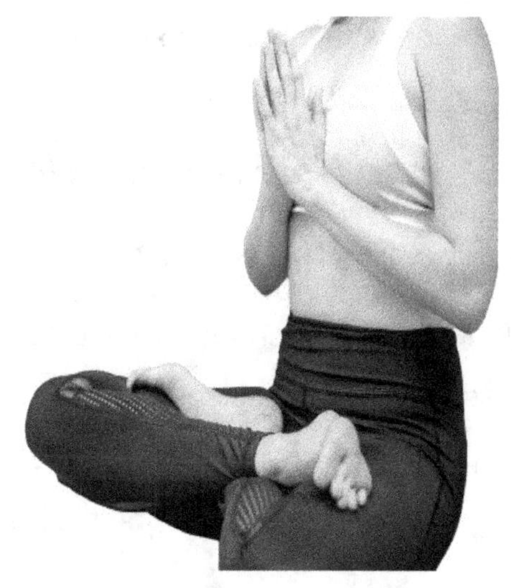

Bodyweight Exercises: Perform exercises such as push-ups, squats, lunges, and planks without the use of equipment to develop strength, flexibility, and muscular tone.

Low-impact exercises, such as walking, cycling, or utilizing an elliptical machine, can provide cardiovascular benefits while putting less strain on the joints.

Remember to listen to your body and select exercises that you enjoy and can maintain in the long run. Consult a certified trainer to create a personalized workout plan based on your fitness level and goals.

III. How To Schedule Workouts During Fasting Period.

Working out during an intermittent fasting phase needs precise planning in order to maximize energy levels and performance. Here are some pointers to help you plan your workouts properly while practicing intermittent fasting:

Select the right fasting window: Choose a fasting window that corresponds to your training plan. For example, you could pick a fasting window that ends immediately before or after your workout.

Time your meals carefully: If you prefer to eat before your workout, schedule your meals such that your last meal is consumed within a reasonable time range before your workout. This will guarantee that you have enough energy without feeling overly full or experiencing discomfort while exercising.

Modify workout intensity: Because intermittent fasting might have an impact on your energy levels, pay attention to your body and modify your workout intensity as needed. High-intensity workouts may be more difficult to complete during fasting times, so consider incorporating more moderate-intensity exercises or focusing on strength training.

Include pre-exercise fuel: If you struggle with energy levels before your workout while fasting, consider incorporating some pre-workout fuel. This can be a modest snack containing carbs and protein, such as a banana with a dollop of nut butter, a handful of nuts, or a protein smoothie. To avoid breaking your fast, keep the portion small.

Post-exercise nutrition: Prioritize refueling your body with a nutritious meal that includes a balance of protein, carbohydrates, and fats after your workout

COMMON CHALLENGES AND HOW TO OVERCOME PLATEAUS AND STALLS

I. Common Challenges Encountered During Intermittent Fasting.

While intermittent fasting has various advantages, there are some common challenges that people may face when using this eating pattern.

Hunger and cravings: Fasting for an extended period of time might cause increased hunger and cravings, especially at the beginning. Your body may need time to acclimatize to the new dietary pattern.

Energy levels and fatigue: Some people may experience a decline in energy levels and feelings of fatigue during fasting. This is especially obvious in the early stages of fasting. It may take some time for the body to acclimatize and use alternative energy sources like stored fat.

Consistency and compliance: Sticking to the designated fasting and eating hours might be difficult, especially when social engagements, various commitments, travel, or unexpected situations arise. It requires a certain amount of commitment and obedience to the fasting and eating times. Maintaining discipline and planning ahead of time can help you overcome this obstacle.

Nutritional deficiencies: Depending on the fasting schedule and food choices, maintaining proper intake of vital elements such as vitamins, minerals, and fiber can be difficult. This difficulty can be reduced by making mindful food choices during eating windows and selecting nutrient-dense options.

Digestive issues: When beginning intermittent fasting, some people may experience digestive problems, such as bloating or constipation.

Your digestive system may need some time to acclimatize to the new food schedule.

Disruption of social activities: Fasting times can interfere with social engagements including food, making participation difficult or finding suitable substitutes difficult. Open communication with friends and family, as well as seeking supporting social networks, can assist with fixing this issue.

Influence on workout performance: Intermittent fasting may impair exercise performance, especially if you work out hard during the fasting phase. Coordination of exercises and meal times can be difficult and may have an impact on performance during training sessions. Experimenting with different fasting and exercise routines might help you discover a healthy balance.

Emotional and psychological aspects: When transitioning to intermittent fasting, some people may experience mood swings, anger, or emotional shifts, as well as feelings of guilt, worry, or compulsive thoughts about food. Being aware of these possible effects and caring for your mental health can be beneficial.

II. Celebrating Your Successes.

Congratulations on overcoming your intermittent fasting challenges! Celebrating your accomplishments is an important part of staying motivated and devoted to your goals. Here are some suggestions for celebrating your successes;

Reward yourself with a nutritious treat: Enjoy a tasty lunch or snack that is in line with your dietary goals. Prepare a nutritious and filling lunch with fresh ingredients, or treat yourself to a healthy dessert.

Have a cheat meal: Allow yourself to enjoy a favorite dish that you've been yearning for, even if it's not part of your typical fasting diet. It's important to create a balance between discipline and fun.

Plan a social gathering: Gather your friends or family to celebrate your successes. You can organize a potluck or go out to a place that caters to your fasting choices.

Take care of yourself: Give yourself a spa day, a massage, or any other sort of self-care you enjoy. It's a terrific way to unwind and reward yourself for your dedication to intermittent fasting.

Reflect and journal: Spend some time reflecting on what you experienced with intermittent fasting. Make a list of your accomplishments, obstacles you faced, and how you feel about your growth. Journaling can be an excellent approach to appreciate and recognize your achievements.

Share your success: Share your achievements with friends, family, or members of a supportive community. Celebrate your victory with people who have supported you and offer encouragement to others who may be suffering similar difficulties.

Remember that how you celebrate your success is entirely up to you. Choose activities that you enjoy and that contribute to your general well-being. Because intermittent fasting is a long-term lifestyle change, it's critical to find healthy and sustainable ways to recognize and celebrate your accomplishments along the way.

Buy something special: Purchase an item or indulge in an activity that you've been wanting for a long time. It could be a new wardrobe, a book, a gadget, or concert or event tickets.

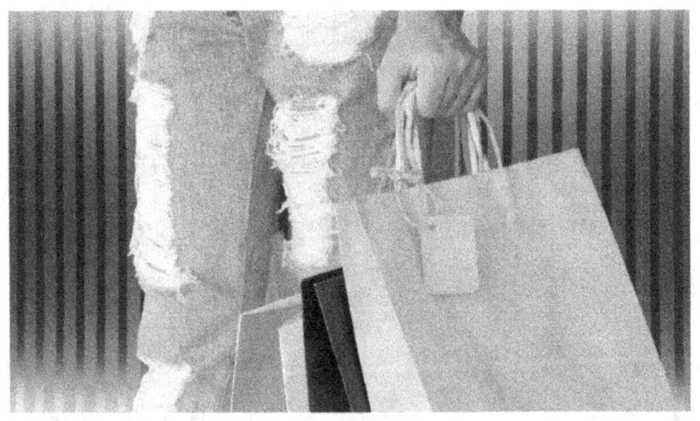

CONCLUSION

In conclusion, "Intermittent Fasting for Women Over 50" offers a comprehensive and clear evaluation of an effective nutritional approach for women in their prime years. This book provides women with the knowledge and resources they need to harness the benefits of intermittent fasting and maximize their health and well-being through a combination of scientific data, practical advice, and inspiring success stories.

One of the book's core strengths is its attention to the special demands and issues that women over 50 encounter. Recognizing the particular hormonal changes and metabolic alterations that occur during this period of life, I have provided specialized information to assist women in safely and efficiently navigating intermittent fasting.

By addressing issues such as bone health, menopause, and muscle upkeep, this book informs women to accept intermittent fasting as a valuable tool for weight control, disease prevention, and healthy aging.

Exploring concerns like autophagy, insulin sensitivity, and hormonal balance, I'd like to think I've demystified the mechanisms behind intermittent fasting and emphasized its potential to improve longevity and vitality. By providing readers with this information, I hope to inspire confidence in this approach as well as offer a thorough grasp of its benefits.

"Intermittent Fasting for Women Over 50" provides practical advice and tactics for successfully implementing intermittent fasting. It addresses common issues and challenges such as hunger management and dealing with social situations.

The book promotes a flexible and personalized approach, acknowledging that each woman's journey is unique. I've helped readers establish a sustainable and enjoyable fasting regimen that matches their lifestyle and goals by providing numerous intermittent fasting protocols and emphasizing the need of self-care.

Finally, "Intermittent Fasting for Women Over 50" is a useful resource that enables women in this age range to take charge of their health and adopt a lifestyle that promotes longevity and vitality.

Sample Meal Plans For Different Types Of Intermittent Fasting.

16:8 Fasting Schedule

7:00 AM	Wake up
7:30 AM	Warm Lemon Honey Water
7:45 AM	Continue Fasting
12:00 PM	Lunch: Avocado/Toast Eggs/Oatmeal OR Bagel/Cheese/Greek Yoghurt and Sunflower seeds.
3:00 PM	Snack: Fruits or Nuts (Apples, Oranges, Peaches, Kiwi, Almonds,Pistachios)
6:00 PM	Dinner: Sautéed chicken breast with Pasta and Banana smoothie OR Cauliflower rice with Orange juice.
7:30 PM	Snack: Vegetable/Fruit Salad OR Smoothies OR Nuts.
8:00 PM	Begin 16 hours Fast.

5:2 Fasting Schedule

Day 1	Eat Normally
Day 2	24 hours Fast
Day 3	Eat Normally
Day 4	Eat Normally
Day 5	24 hours Fast
Day 6	Eat Normally
Day 7	Eat Normally

List of meals to help you decide what to eat.

- Whole Wheat Pancake with Coconut Creamer.
- Oatmeal with fried Eggs and Rashers Bacon.
- Seeds Crackers with cream Cheese and mushroom.
- Omelette with Chorizo, Mushrooms.

- Yogurt with seeds and nuts.
- Fatty biltong with Chicken Salad.
- Creamed Spinach, roasted vegetables with cauliflower rice.
- Pork Rashers with Quinoa and Sauteed Vegetables.
- Chicken stir-fried in Olive oil with Carrots, Spinach and baby corn.
- Fried Fish with Salad, Cheddar mushroom, Tomatoes and Lettuce.
- Cauliflower base Pizza with mushrooms and Tomato Puree.
- Meatloaf stuffed with Sautéed Spinach and Cream Cheese.
- Mashed Potatoes with Sautéed Chicken breast and sweet corn.

Protein

Meat

- Chicken
- Turkey
- Beef
- Egg
- Sausage
- Bacon
- Pork
- Mutton

Seafood

- Shrimp
- Tuna
- Salmon
- Mackerel
- Cod, Tilapia
- Scallop
- Crab, Clam
- Snail, Periwinkles

Vegetables

- Asparagus
- Broccoli
- Cauliflower
- Brussel Sprouts
- Carrots
- Cabbage
- Spinach
- Green Beans
- Egg plants
- Cucumber
- Bell peppers
- Onion, Garlic
- Potatoes
- Kale
- Lettuce
- Beets

Fruits

- Apples
- Pineapple
- Oranges
- Lemon/Lime
- Grapes
- Plums
- Apricot
- Peaches
- Berries
- Cherries
- Kiwi
- Bananas
- Watermelon
- Pears
- Mangoes

These fruits can be eaten whole or blended into smoothies or fruit juice.

Nuts and Seeds

- Cashew nuts

- Almond
- Walnuts
- Pecans
- Pistachios
- Sunflower seeds
- Flax seeds
- Chia seeds
- Sesame seeds
- Pumpkin seeds

Whole Grains

- Quinoa
- Rice
- Pasta
- Oats
- Corn

www.ingramcontent.com/pod-product-compliance
Lightning Source LLC
Chambersburg PA
CBHW061520250726
48657CB00005B/1982